TWO SISTERS PUBLISHING

Skincare Renewal

A Practical Guide for Women Over 50 to Achieve Refined, Glowing, and Hydrated Skin in only 10 Minutes a Day.

"Happiness is a habit. So is your skincare."

LINDEN TYLER

Contents

1

Introduction

Are you searching for ways to make your skin look better but are not sure where to start? Likely you've tried lots of different skin tips and still haven't found the right answer. This guide is for women who, like me, have crossed the fabulous fifty mark. Our skin doesn't quite bounce back like it used to and we are noticing!

I'm Kim - think of this book as a conversation between friends on the path to better skin - let's go! I have tried many different skin creams and routines. Some worked and some did not. I love skincare and in this book I share the basics to restart a self-care routine or refresh your current one.

This book will help you learn simple, quick steps that can help your skin in 10 minutes a day. We'll talk about how to make a daily skincare routine that is practical and fits into your life. The chapters will explain more about products you are familiar with and others you have not tried yet.

We'll also look at how small changes to daily habits can add up to big results for your skin. Yet, I can't promise your skin will change overnight by simply reading my book. I give practical information but only you can put a routine in place to gain renewed skin.

Yes, over the age of 50, our skin has transformations that can be challenging. Let this be an opportunity to meet your ever-evolving self with confidence and grace.

2

Your Changing Skin

As we journey into our fifties and beyond, our skin tells the story of our lives. It's not about aging; it's about living. Embrace these changes while finding ways to nurture and revitalize your skin. Self-care isn't a trend; it's an essential practice that helps us look and feel our best. A consistent skincare routine can improve concerns that many women over 50 experience.

Lines and Wrinkles

Lines and wrinkles are often caused by the natural decrease in collagen and elastin in our skin. To help reduce these, focus on products that boost hydration and firmness. Ingredients like hyaluronic acid, which retains moisture, and retinoids that stimulate collagen production. Lines and wrinkles are more than marks on our skin, yet we can feel self-conscious. Using the right products can reduce signs of aging around the eyes, mouth, and forehead.

To smooth and hydrate lines, focus on ingredients known for anti-aging properties. Hyaluronic acid is a hydrator that can hold up to 1000 times its weight in water! It is best known for plumping the skin and smoothing out fine lines. When applied to damp skin and sealed in with a richer cream or oil, it becomes a staple for any anti-aging routine.

- A retinoid cream can help to reduce the appearance of wrinkles and improve skin texture. A prescription-strength cream several times a week can benefit areas of your face and neck where movement may deepen lines. Be aware that retinoids can be drying. It is important to balance their use with hydrating ingredients. Start slowly to build your tolerance.
- Peptides are also vital. The amino acid chains in peptides help to signal the skin to produce more collagen and elastin. These two proteins are crucial for maintaining the skin's structure and elasticity. Apply a peptide serum under a moisturizer to firm the skin and reduce the visibility of wrinkles

Look for eye creams with added antioxidants like vitamin C or E to protect this sensitive area. Vitamin C can also help brighten the skin, reducing the dullness that can go with aging skin.

Additionally, lifestyle factors such as adequate hydration, a balanced diet rich in antioxidants, and sun protection are indispensable. Wearing sunglasses to avoid squinting and applying a broad-spectrum SPF daily will help prevent new wrinkles from forming and protect against worsening existing ones.

For those seeking a more intensive treatment, professional options like laser therapy, micro-needling, or chemical peels can provide more dramatic results. Under the guidance of a dermatologist these treatments can help reduce the depth and appearance of wrinkles by encouraging deeper collagen production.

By incorporating these targeted treatments and maintaining a routine tailored to combat lines and wrinkles, you can achieve a smoother, more youthful complexion. This dedicated approach not only addresses the existing signs of aging but also provides a preventive measure to maintain your skin's health and vibrancy.

Types of Skin: Dry, Oily, or Combination

Changes in hormone levels can leave us with dry, oily, or even combination skin. Understanding your skin type is crucial in selecting the right products. For dry skin, creams rich in fatty acids and ceramides can help rebuild the skin's barrier. Oily skin benefits from lightweight, water-based moisturizers and non-comedogenic products that won't clog pores. Those with combination skin might need to use different products on different areas of the face to balance the skin's needs.

Understanding your skin type is crucial to selecting the right skincare and makeup products that will work best for you. As our skin matures, it may change what worked in the past and not be as effective now. Here's how to identify and care for dry, oily, or combination skin, along with makeup tips for each type.

Dry Skin

Dry skin often feels tight and may show signs of flaking and redness. An underproduction of natural oils leads to a compromised skin barrier. For dry skin, look for hydrating serums and rich moisturizers that contain ingredients like hyaluronic acid, glycerin, and ceramides. These help to lock in moisture and repair the skin's natural barrier. Night creams with oils such as argan or jojoba can also be beneficial as they provide an extra moisture boost overnight.

When it comes to makeup, liquid or cream foundations that have a hydrating formula work best for dry skin. These foundations help to prevent clumping on dry patches and give the skin a dewy glow. Avoid powder foundations as they can absorb moisture and dry out areas.

Oily Skin

Oily skin appears shiny, especially in the T-zone (forehead, nose, and chin), and may be prone to breakouts. This skin type produces excess sebum, which can clog pores. For oily skin, use lightweight, water-based products and non-comedogenic moisturizers to hydrate the skin without adding extra oil. Products containing salicylic acid or benzoyl peroxide can help manage acne and control oil production.

The best foundation for oily skin is an oil-free, matte-finish liquid foundation or mineral powder foundation. These formulations help to absorb excess oil and shine throughout the day, maintaining a smooth, matte finish.

Combination Skin

Combination skin means you might have areas that are both oily and dry. Usually, the T-zone is oily, while the cheeks, jawline, and eye area might be dry. This skin type benefits from using different products tailored to specific areas. A balanced approach with a lightweight, hydrating serum for dry areas and a mattifying moisturizer for oily zones can work well.

For combination skin, using a primer can help to balance the skin's different needs before applying makeup. A liquid foundation that has a natural or satin finish is generally suitable, as it can provide hydration without contributing to oiliness. In some cases, applying a light dusting of powder in the oily areas can help to set the foundation and control shine. By identifying your skin type and choosing products and makeup that cater to its unique needs, you can achieve a balanced, healthy-looking complexion. Assessing your skin's condition and adjusting your routine as needed will help maintain its best state as it changes with age.

Dark Spots and Hyperpigmentation

Dark spots, or hyperpigmentation, are often the result of long-term sun exposure. They can also become more noticeable as the skin's natural ability to fight UV damage weakens with age. To combat this, use products containing vitamin C, which brightens the complexion, and sunscreens with high SPF to prevent further pigmentation. Regular use of exfoliating products like alpha hydroxy acids (AHAs) can also help fade these spots over time. As we age, our skin often shows texture changes such as roughness, dry patches, or crepey skin. The cause of these conditions are a combination of sun exposure, hormonal changes you may experience during menopause, and environmental stressors.

How It Happens

Dark spots, also known as age spots, are the result of prolonged exposure to UV rays which stimulate melanocytes, the melanin-producing cells in the skin. Over time, these cells can overproduce melanin in certain areas, leading to visible dark patches. Hyperpigmentation can occur from acne scars or through hormonal changes that trigger an increase in melanin.

Topical Creams and Treatments

To reduce the appearance of dark spots and uneven skin texture, topical treatments that include ingredients like hydroquinone, kojic acid, and vitamin C are effective. Hydroquinone works by decreasing the production and increasing the breakdown of melanin pigments in the skin. Kojic acid also inhibits melanin production and is a good alternative for those who might be sensitive to hydroquinone.

Retinoids can help with texture issues by promoting cell turnover and collagen production, smoothing the skin and reducing the appearance of dark spots over time. Alpha hydroxy acids (AHAs), like glycolic acid, are another option to help exfoliate the skin, remove dead skin cells, and brighten the complexion.

By combining the right skincare products with healthy lifestyle habits, you can reduce the appearance of dark spots, hyperpigmentation, and texture changes. These efforts help maintain your skin's natural beauty and resilience against the visible signs of aging.

Sagging Skin

Sagging skin is another common concern due to the loss of skin's natural elasticity. To counteract this, look for products that contain peptides and antioxidants. These ingredients help to firm and lift the skin. Performing facial exercises and massaging your face can also promote blood flow and tighten the skin, enhancing the effects of your skincare products.

Sagging skin is a common concern among women over 50, resulting from the natural decrease in collagen and elastin production as we age. There are several non-invasive ways to improve the appearance of sagging skin, at home or in a professional setting.

- **Light Therapy**: Light therapy, especially red light therapy, is an excellent tool for tightening sagging skin. It works by using low-level wavelengths of light to stimulate collagen production, reducing wrinkles and enhancing skin firmness. Red light therapy devices are available for home use or in a spa setting.

- **Facial Massage**: Engaging in face massage is another effective method to combat sagging skin. This practice involves performing specific facial exercises that target the muscles of the face, improving blood circulation and promoting the tightening of skin. Regular practice can lead to noticeable improvements in the firmness and tone of your facial skin.
- **Jade Roller**: Using a jade roller can help improve the elasticity of the skin and promote lymphatic drainage. Rolling it across the face can reduce puffiness, tone the skin, and encourage detoxification. For an enhanced effect, keep the jade roller in the refrigerator before use to add a cooling effect that tightens pores and firms the skin.
- **Professional Spa Treatments**: Many spas offer non-invasive treatments designed to tighten sagging skin. Services such as microcurrent facials, which use low-level electrical currents to stimulate the facial muscles and skin cells, are popular. These treatments can improve skin texture and elasticity without the need for surgical procedures.
- **Regular Moisturizing and Proper Nutrition**: Incorporating a rich moisturizing routine and maintaining a diet rich in antioxidants and healthy fats can also support skin health. Moisturizers with ingredients like hyaluronic acid can provide the skin with necessary hydration, while a balanced diet sustains skin repair and collagen production.

By integrating these techniques and treatments into your skincare routine, you can improve the appearance of sagging skin. Each of these options offers a gentle, relaxing way to care for your skin while combating the signs of aging.

Dark Under-Eye Circles and Puffiness

Dark circles under the eyes can make you look more tired than you feel. These are often caused by thinning skin and loss of fat and collagen and make the reddish-blue blood vessels under your eyes more noticeable. A dedicated eye cream with caffeine can help constrict blood vessels, reducing their visibility. Eye creams with peptides can also restore thickness to the skin, helping to hide dark circles.

- **Targeted Creams and Serums**: Look for eye creams and serums rich in vitamin C, caffeine, and retinol. Vitamin C helps to brighten the under-eye area, while caffeine reduces puffiness by constricting blood vessels, and retinol promotes collagen production to improve the skin's elasticity. Products containing peptides or hyaluronic acid are also beneficial as they hydrate and plump the skin
- **Tools and non-invasive services**: A jade roller massages the eye area, promoting lymphatic drainage and reducing puffiness. This tool is most effective when used with a cooled serum or cream for added anti-inflammatory effects. Professional treatments like LED light therapy and lymphatic drainage massages offered at spas can also help reduce under-eye puffiness and dark circles.
- **Instant Puffiness Reducers**: Products designed to reduce puffiness often contain ingredients like witch hazel or caffeine. The applied serum or gel works by tightening and cooling the skin, providing temporary relief from puffiness. Such products are particularly useful for mornings when you need to look refreshed.

Lack of Elasticity and Loss of Collagen

As our skin's elasticity decreases, it may begin to feel less firm. To improve elasticity, focus on hydration and nutrients that support skin health. Ingredients like collagen, elastin, and omega fatty acids can help strengthen the skin's structure. Your skin may appear more youthful and resilient.

Why It Happens

Collagen and elastin are proteins responsible for the skin's structure and elasticity. As you age, your body's production of these proteins decreases due to factors like genetic aging, environmental exposure (such as UV light), and lifestyle choices (like smoking or poor diet). Hormonal changes during menopause also contribute to a decrease in collagen, exacerbating skin aging.

Slowing the Process

To slow the reduction of elasticity and collagen, incorporate a few key practices into your daily routine:

- **Sun Protection**: Regular use of sunscreen with at least SPF 30 can protect the skin from UV damage, one of the primary causes of collagen breakdown.
- **Healthy Diet**: Eating foods rich in antioxidants, vitamins (especially Vitamin C and E), and omega-3 fatty acids can help protect and replenish skin cells. Vitamin C is particularly important for collagen synthesis.
- **Skincare Regimen**: Products containing retinoids, peptides, and antioxidants can support collagen production. Retinoids speed up cell turnover and increase collagen synthesis, while peptides act as building blocks for proteins in the skin.
- **Hydration**: Keeping the skin hydrated with hyaluronic acid, which can hold up to 1000 times its weight in water, helps maintain skin plumpness and elasticity.
- **Supplements**: Consult a medical professional for advice on consuming dietary supplements known to boost collagen levels. Collagen peptides in powder form are popular and can be added to drinks or food. Supplements containing hyaluronic acid, Vitamin C, and amino acids also support skin health and collagen production.

- **Topical Products**: Look for serums and creams designed to boost collagen and elastin in the skin. These often contain hyaluronic acid, retinol, and Vitamin C. Applying these products can help improve the skin's firmness and reduce the appearance of fine lines and wrinkles.

By understanding and addressing the loss of elasticity and collagen, you can take effective steps to maintain healthier, more resilient skin. Regular use of appropriate skincare products, along with protective and nutritive measures, can diminish the impact of aging on your skin's appearance.

3

Skincare Products

Cleanser

Starting your skincare routine with the right cleanser sets the stage for every other product you apply. Cleansers remove dirt, oil, and impurities from your skin, preparing it for the next steps in your skincare regimen. Depending on your skin type, you might choose a gel cleanser for oily skin, a cream-based cleanser for dry skin, or a balancing cleanser for combination skin. If your skin is particularly sensitive, look for gentle formulas that are free from harsh chemicals and fragrances.

Cleansers impact the health and appearance of skin. It's not about removing makeup; a good cleanser will also help to manage skin problems such as acne, dryness, and excessive oiliness.

Types of Cleansers

- **Gel Cleansers**: These are clear and have a gel-like consistency. They are particularly effective for deep cleaning and are best suited for oily and combination skin types. Gel cleansers work well to unclog pores, remove excess oil, and kill bacteria that may lead to acne.

- **Cream Cleansers**: Cream-based cleansers are richer and offer more hydration, making them ideal for dry or sensitive skin types. They cleanse the skin without stripping it of its natural oils, providing a soothing and nourishing effect that helps to maintain the skin's moisture barrier.
- **Foaming Cleansers**: Perfect for combination skin, foaming cleansers are a versatile option that can address both dry and oily patches. They lather up and remove impurities without stripping the skin.
- **Oil Cleansers**: These can work for all skin types but are beneficial for dry skin. Oil cleansers dissolve makeup and impurities while moisturizing the skin but without over-drying it.
- **Micellar Water**: A gentle option for all skin types, particularly sensitive or acne-prone skin. Micellar water uses tiny micelles (oil molecules) that attract and sweep away dirt and oil, without irritating the skin.

Cleansing both in the morning and at night is essential. In the morning, cleansing helps remove any toxins the skin eliminates during the night and prepares the skin for other skincare products and makeup. At night, it removes makeup and the buildup of oil and dirt from the day, which can contribute to acne and dull skin if not cleaned away.

Understanding and choosing the right type of cleanser for your skin type can ensure skin is clean, clear, and ready to absorb other products, paving the way for healthier skin without stripping it of its natural oils.

Toner

Toners are often misunderstood but are essential for restoring the skin's pH balance after cleansing. For oily skin, a clarifying toner with ingredients like salicylic acid can help reduce the appearance of pores and control excess oil. For dry or sensitive skin, a hydrating toner with soothing agents like aloe vera or rose water can add a layer of moisture and calm the skin. Applying toner with a soft cotton pad can additionally help in exfoliating the surface of your skin, making it ready for the serums and moisturizers that follow.

Purpose of Skin Toner

- **Removes Residue**: Even after cleansing, impurities and traces of makeup can remain. Toner helps remove these completely, ensuring the skin is clean.
- **Balances pH**: Skin has an acidic pH, and cleansing can disturb this balance. Toner helps to restore the skin to its natural pH, enhancing its barrier function and health.
- **Hydrates and Refreshes**: Many toners contain hydrating ingredients that help to moisturize the skin and refresh it, leaving it smooth and soft.
- **Prepares Skin**: By balancing and hydrating, toners prepare the skin to more absorb the active ingredients in serums and moisturizers.

When to Use Toner

Apply toner after cleansing and before serums or moisturizers. Use it as part of both morning and evening skincare routines to maximize its benefits.

Best Types of Toner for Each Skin Type

- **Dry Skin**: Look for hydrating toners that contain ingredients like glycerin, hyaluronic acid, or rosewater. These ingredients help to lock in moisture and soothe dry, tight skin.

- **Oily Skin**: Toners with ingredients such as witch hazel, tea tree oil, or salicylic acid can help to manage excess oil production, reduce pores, and prevent breakouts.
- **Combination Skin**: A balancing toner that addresses both dry and oily areas is ideal. Ingredients like chamomile or green tea can soothe the skin while managing oiliness in the T-zone.
- **Sensitive Skin**: Choose toners that are free of alcohol and fragrances and contain soothing ingredients like aloe vera or cucumber. These gentle formulas help to calm irritation and reduce redness without over-stripping the skin.

Incorporating the right type of toner into your skincare routine can enhance the health and appearance of your skin, making it a crucial step for anyone looking to achieve a clear, balanced, and hydrated complexion.

Facial Serums

Serums target specific skincare concerns thanks to their potent active ingredients. A facial serum is a lightweight moisturizer that penetrates deeper to deliver active ingredients into your skin. They address a variety of issues, from aging and wrinkles to dullness and hyperpigmentation. Choose a serum based on what your skin needs most: antioxidants like vitamin C for protection against environmental damage, hyaluronic acid for hydration, or retinoids for anti-aging properties. Apply your serum after toning but before moisturizing to ensure its active ingredients penetrate the skin.

Purpose of Facial Serum

- **Concentrated Care**: Serums deliver high concentrations of specific active ingredients to the skin. This is beneficial for addressing targeted concerns such as aging, hyperpigmentation, or dullness.

- **Enhanced Absorption**: Their light and thin consistency absorb and penetrate skin more than traditional moisturizers
- **Customization**: The variety of serums available allows women to tailor routines to specific skin needs and concerns.

Why It Is Important

Using a serum is crucial because of its ability to act at a deeper level and its efficiency in delivering potent ingredients to the skin. This can enhance the health and appearance of the skin, making serums a vital step in both preventive and corrective skincare regimens.

When to Use Facial Serum

Serums applied after cleansing and toning but before moisturizing ensures the potent ingredients can penetrate skin before applying creams. For best results, use serums twice daily, during both morning and evening skincare routines.

Best Types of Serum for Each Skin Type

- **Dry Skin**: Look for hydrating serums that contain ingredients like hyaluronic acid, glycerin, or Vitamin E. These ingredients help attract and lock in moisture, reducing dryness and making the skin appear smoother and plumper.
- **Oily Skin**: Serums with niacinamide, salicylic acid, or zinc can help regulate oil production, reduce pore size, and clear out clogged pores, leading to clearer and less greasy skin.
- **Combination Skin**: A serum that balances hydration and oil control is ideal. Ingredients like hyaluronic acid combined with green tea or lavender can hydrate the skin while controlling shiny

areas, particularly in the T-zone.

- **Sensitive Skin**: Serums formulated with soothing ingredients like aloe vera, chamomile, or oat extract can calm inflammation and redness.
- **Aging Skin**: Anti-aging serums that contain antioxidants like Vitamin C, retinol, or peptides are beneficial as they stimulate collagen production, fight free radicals, and improve the skin's firmness and elasticity.

Integrating the right serum into your skincare routine can elevate your regimen, providing targeted treatment and boosting the effectiveness of the products that follow.

Under Eye Cream

The skin under your eyes is thinner and more delicate than the rest of your face, making it more susceptible to signs of aging such as dark circles and puffiness. An under-eye cream can help to address crepey skin you may be seeing. Look for creams with caffeine to reduce puffiness, peptides to boost collagen production, and antioxidants to protect against environmental stressors. Tap the eye cream using your ring finger to apply it without pulling on the delicate skin.

Purpose of Under Eye Cream

- **Hydration:** Under eye creams provide intense moisture to the delicate eye area, helping to reduce dryness and fine lines.
- **Targeting Specific Concerns**: These creams often contain ingredients aimed at reducing dark circles, puffiness, and signs of aging like crow's feet.
- **Protection**: Some under eye creams include ingredients that help protect this sensitive area from environmental stressors like UV

rays and pollution.

Problems Under Eye Cream Helps With

- **Dark Circles**: Ingredients like caffeine and vitamin C can help brighten the under-eye area and reduce the appearance of discoloration.
- **Puffiness**: Cooling agents and anti-inflammatory ingredients such as cucumber extract and peptides can reduce swelling and soothe the under-eye area.
- **Fine Lines and Crepiness**: Hydrating ingredients and those that promote collagen production, such as hyaluronic acid and retinol, can plump the skin and smooth out fine lines.

Importance in a Daily Routine

- **Preventative Care**: Regular use can help prevent the development of fine lines and wrinkles.
- **Intensive Treatment**: Provides targeted treatment to a vulnerable area that other facial moisturizers may not address.
- **Enhanced Appearance**: Consistent use can improve the appearance of the under-eye area, making it look brighter and more youthful.

Results from Using Under Eye Cream

- Reduced appearance of dark circles and puffiness.
- Minimization of fine lines and wrinkles.
- Brighter and more even skin tone around the eyes.

It's important to use under eye cream as part of your morning and evening routines to see these effects. Patience is key, as it can take a few weeks to notice visible improvements.

Pigmentation and Acne Cream

For those with acne-prone or blemish-sensitive skin, a targeted blemish cream can be crucial. These creams generally contain acne-fighting ingredients like benzoyl peroxide or salicylic acid that help to clear existing breakouts and prevent new ones from forming. It's important to apply blemish creams onto cleaned, affected areas to maximize their effectiveness while minimizing irritation to the rest of your skin.

Pigmentation creams address specific concerns such as uneven skin tone, dark spots, rosacea, and acne breakouts. These creams often contain active ingredients that can help reduce these issues and improve the health and appearance of the skin.

Purpose of Pigmentation and Acne Creams

- **Pigmentation Issues**: Creams intended for pigmentation problems often contain ingredients like hydroquinone, kojic acid, or vitamin C, known for their skin-lightening properties. These ingredients help to fade dark spots and even out skin tone.
- **Acne**: Acne creams may include benzoyl peroxide, salicylic acid, or retinoids. These substances help to clear pores, reduce inflammation, and prevent future breakouts.

What to Expect

- **Visible Improvement**: With regular use, these creams can lead to a noticeable reduction in dark spots, redness, and acne. Yet, the effectiveness and speed of results can vary based on the severity of the condition and individual skin type.

- **Consistency is Key**: Many of these products need consistent application over several weeks or even months before seeing significant improvements.

Frequency of Use

- The frequency of these creams should depend on the specific product and skin sensitivity. Some creams are for daily use, while others may need less frequent use, especially those containing stronger active ingredients.
- Follow the usage instructions provided on the product label or by a dermatologist.

Types Available

- **Over-the-Counter Creams**: These are available and can address mild pigmentation and acne issues. They are generally less potent but safer for long-term use.
- **Prescription Creams**: When over-the-counter products do not provide the desired results, prescription creams may be necessary. These have higher concentrations of active ingredients.

Are These Creams Worth Including in a Routine?

Including pigmentation and acne creams in your skincare routine can be very beneficial, especially if you are dealing with specific skin issues that these products target. Remember to:

- Choose the right product for your specific skin concern and use according to the directions to avoid potential skin irritation or damage.

- Consider the potency of the ingredients—stronger isn't always better, particularly for sensitive skin.
- Be patient and consistent with the application to achieve the best results.
- These creams can be a worthwhile investment for enhancing skin appearance and tackling problematic skin conditions.

Daytime Moisturizer

A good day moisturizer not only hydrates your skin but also protects it from the daily aggressors like UV rays and pollution. For dry skin, look for ingredients that lock in moisture like glycerin or hyaluronic acid. If your skin is oily, opt for a lightweight, non-comedogenic moisturizer that won't clog pores. Many day moisturizers also come with SPF protection, which is essential for preventing skin aging and damage.

Purpose of Daytime Moisturizer

Using a daytime moisturizer every day helps maintain the skin's moisture barrier, which is essential for keeping the skin healthy and preventing water loss. Regular use can lead to:

- Improved skin texture and elasticity.
- Reduction in the appearance of fine lines and dry patches.
- Enhanced radiance and a more even skin tone.

Benefits from Continued Use

Using a daytime moisturizer can result in hydrated, resilient skin that looks younger and feels smoother. It also helps in:

- Minimizing skin flakiness and tightness.
- Protecting against environmental damage due to antioxidants and

other protective ingredients.
- Preparing the skin for smoother application of makeup.

Choosing the Right Moisturizer for Your Skin Type

- **Dry Skin**: Look for creams that are rich in emollients and humectants such as hyaluronic acid, glycerin, and ceramides, which help to lock in moisture and repair the skin barrier.
- **Oily Skin**: Opt for lightweight, non-comedogenic formulas that hydrate without adding excess oil. Ingredients like hyaluronic acid or aloe vera provide moisture without clogging pores.
- **Combination Skin**: Choose a moisturizer that balances hydration. Lotions or gels with ingredients like dimethicone, which can hydrate dry areas while not over-moisturizing oily zones, are ideal.

Key Ingredients and Their Percentages

When comparing moisturizers, look for key ingredients that benefit your specific skin concerns:

- **Hyaluronic Acid**: Known for its capacity to hold up to 1000 times its weight in water, making it a top choice for hydration.
- **Niacinamide**: Ideal for both hydrating skin and reducing redness, found in concentrations of 2-5%.
- **Vitamin E**: An antioxidant that protects against free radical damage, often used in concentrations of 0.1-1%.
- **SPF**: Daytime moisturizers should contain SPF 30 or higher to protect the skin from UV rays.

While percentages can give a hint about a product's potency, the formulation is more critical. A well-formulated product with lower percentages of several synergistic ingredients often outperforms a product with a high concentration of one single ingredient. The combination and stability of ingredients are crucial in making a moisturizer effective.Using the right type of daytime moisturizer can improve the health and appearance of your skin, making it an indispensable step in your daily skincare routine.

Nighttime Moisturizer (aka Night or Heavy Cream)

Night creams support skin repair and regeneration while you sleep. They tend to be richer and more hydrating than day creams and may contain ingredients that are best used overnight to avoid sunlight exposure, such as certain retinoids and acids. Choosing a night cream that's right for your skin type can enhance your skin's natural overnight healing process, helping you to wake up with refreshed, softer skin.

By understanding these essential types of skincare products, you can tailor your skincare routines to specific skin needs, achieving better results and maintaining healthier skin.

Night creams are an essential part of an evening skincare routine, designed to support skin repair and rejuvenation while you sleep. They are often richer and more hydrating than daytime moisturizers, hence sometimes referred to as "heavy" creams.

Purpose of Night Cream

The primary function of a night cream is to nourish and repair the skin overnight. During sleep, the skin's blood flow increases, and the organ rebuilds its collagen and repairs damage from UV exposure, reducing wrinkles and age spots. Formulated night creams take advantage of this natural healing process.

Benefits from Continued Use

- Enhance skin's firmness and elasticity.
- Reduce the appearance of fine lines and wrinkles.
- Provide deep hydration and intense nourishment.
- Promote a more even skin tone and texture.

Usage Recommendations

- Apply night cream every evening as part of your skincare routine.
- At least 30 minutes before bedtime to ensure it absorbs and doesn't transfer to your pillow.
- Apply your night cream over any serums or treatments but under any oils. The active ingredients penetrate without the denser texture of an oil blocking it.

Choosing the Right Night Cream for Your Skin Type

- **Dry Skin**: Look for night creams with ingredients like shea butter, plant oils (like argan or jojoba oil), and ceramides that provide deep hydration and help restore the skin's barrier.
- **Oily Skin**: Choose non-comedogenic formulas that hydrate and repair without causing breakouts. Ingredients like glycolic acid and retinoids can be beneficial as they help reduce oil production and clear pores.
- **Combination Skin**: Opt for a balancing cream with hyaluronic acid that provides moisture where needed without overwhelming oily areas.

Key Ingredients and Their Percentages

- **Retinol**: Helps in skin cell turnover and collagen synthesis, found in concentrations from 0.01% to 1%.

- **Peptides**: Support skin repair and firmness, used in varying concentrations depending on the product.
- **Antioxidants (like Vitamin C and E)**: Help fight free radical damage, usually around 0.1% to 3%.
- **Hyaluronic Acid**: Provides deep hydration, effective at 0.5% to 2%.

A well-formulated night cream will hydrate and deliver active ingredients that help improve skin concerns specific to your skin type. The consistency and richness of a night cream are pivotal in ensuring that your skin remains supported in its natural overnight recovery processes.

4

Developing a Routine

Establishing a skincare routine that is both achievable and sustainable is crucial to maintain and enhance skin health. The key to success lies in simplicity and consistency, ensuring that the routine fits into daily life. I will outline a 5-minute morning routine and a 5-minute evening routine, designed to be straightforward, yet effective, facilitating a higher likelihood of adherence and success.

5 Minute Morning Routine

A 5-minute morning routine is all you need to kickstart your day on the right note, ensuring your skin feels refreshed and protected without demanding too much time. The routine is simple and efficient, which makes it easy to stick to, ensuring consistency—the real secret to seeing lasting benefits.

- **Cleansing (1 minute)**: Start your day with a hydrating cleanser to remove any traces of night creams and natural oils accumulated overnight but doesn't strip the skin of its natural oils. A quick, thorough wash helps to prepare your skin for the next steps in your routine.

- **Applying Toner (1 minute)**: After cleansing apply a gentle alcohol-free toner to balance the skin's pH and refine pores. This step also prepares your skin for better absorption of the products that follow.
- **Serum Application (1 minute)**: Use a serum that targets specific concerns such as hydration, brightening, or anti-aging. For a morning routine, vitamin C serums are excellent for their brightening properties and ability to fight free radicals. Apply a few drops to your fingertips and press into the skin for quick absorption.
- **Moisturizing and Sun Protection (2 minutes)**: Finish off with a moisturizer that includes SPF, or apply moisturizer first and then a separate sunscreen. This step is crucial as it hydrates your skin while also protecting it from harmful UV rays. Choose a product with at least SPF 30 to ensure adequate protection.

Remember, the key to this routine is consistency. It's more beneficial to follow a simple routine every day than to attempt a complex regimen that you cannot maintain. Set your skincare products in a visible and accessible spot in your bathroom to remind you of your routine each morning. This visibility acts as a prompt and streamlines your process, making it easier to commit to your skincare every morning.

5-Minute Evening Routine

Ending your day with a concise, 5-minute evening routine is not only a great way to unwind but also crucial for preparing your skin for its overnight recovery process. This simple routine ensures that you give your skin the attention it needs to repair and rejuvenate, setting the stage for a glowing complexion.

- **Cleansing and Toning (1 minute)**: Your evening cleanse is the most important step of the day. It removes makeup, dirt, and pollutants that have accumulated on your skin. Consider a double cleanse if you wear makeup or sunscreen, first using an oil-based cleanser to break down products, followed by your regular cleanser to clean the skin. Use a gentle, alcohol-free toner to remove any residual impurities and tone the skin.

- **Night Serum or Treatment (2 minutes)**: Evening is the ideal time to apply targeted treatments like retinoids or peptides, which can work overnight to increase cell turnover, improve skin texture and support collagen production. If new to retinoids, start to build tolerance. After cleansing, apply a treatment that targets specific concerns focusing on areas that need the most attention, like wrinkles and dark spots.

- **Moisturize (1 minute)**: Hydration is key, especially at night when your skin undergoes most of its healing and regenerating processes. Use a richer moisturizer than you do in the morning to nourish and hydrate the skin . Look for ingredients like hyaluronic acid, which can help lock in moisture, and ceramides, which strengthen the skin barrier.

- **Eye Cream (1 minute)**: Don't forget to apply an eye cream as part of your evening routine. The skin around your eyes is thinner and more delicate, making it more prone to dryness, dark circles, puffiness, and fine lines. A targeted eye cream can help moisturize and repair this sensitive area overnight.

To ensure consistency with your evening routine, keep your nighttime skincare products together in one place, making them easy to access each evening. You might also find it helpful to set a reminder on your phone or maintain a skincare journal to track your routine and any changes in your skin's condition.

By adhering to these two simple 5-minute routines, you establish a consistent skincare practice that not only addresses immediate skin concerns but also lays the foundation for long-term skin health and vitality. As comfort with the routine grows, it can expand with extra steps or specialized treatments as desired.

5

Supporting Your Skin

Maintaining healthy skin, especially after 50, goes beyond applying the right products in the morning and evening. It involves adopting a holistic approach to your daily life. The actions you take throughout the day impact your skin's health and appearance.

Getting Better Quality of Sleep

Sleep is a critical component of skin health. It's during sleep that your body repairs itself — this includes your skin. Improved sleep quality enhances your skin's ability to renew and recover from daily stressors such as UV exposure and pollution. Sleep isn't only a period of rest; it's a time for the body's repair processes. Getting enough quality sleep each night is essential for maintaining vibrant skin, health, and well-being. Aim for 7-8 hours of sleep per night to allow your body and skin to recover and regenerate.

Tips for Better Sleep

- Establish a consistent bedtime and wake-up time.
- Create a restful environment in your bedroom, which may include

blackout curtains, comfortable bedding, and a cooler temperature.
- Avoid stimulants like caffeine and screen time at least an hour before bed.

Optimal Sleep Timing

Research suggests that the best time to sleep to align with natural circadian rhythms (your body's internal clock) is to go to bed between 10 PM and 11 PM and wake up between 6 AM and 7 AM. This timing helps maximize the quality of sleep, including the amount of restorative REM sleep you receive.

Tips for Achieving Quality Sleep

- **Establish a Routine**: Going to bed and waking up at the same time every day sets your body's internal clock to expect sleep at a certain time night after night.
- **Temperature**: Keep your bedroom cool to lower your body temperature for sleep.
- **Lighting**: Use blackout curtains or an eye mask to block out light, making it easier to fall asleep and stay asleep.
- **Noise**: Consider a white noise machine or a fan to drown out disturbing sounds. Consistent, soft noise can help soothe you to sleep.
- **Essential Oils**: Scents like lavender or chamomile can be relaxing. Use these in a diffuser or as a part of your nighttime skincare routine.
- **Relaxing Activities**: Engage in calming activities such as reading a book or practicing meditation to wind down before bed.
- **Avoid Electronics**: Turn off electronic devices at least an hour before bedtime to reduce blue light exposure, which can disrupt your sleep cycle.

- **Clothing**: Wear light, breathable nightclothes to prevent overheating.
- **Bedding**: Use a satin pillowcase, which is gentler on the skin and hair, and invest in comfortable, supportive mattresses and pillows.

By incorporating these practices into your nighttime routine, you can enhance the quality of your sleep, leading to noticeable improvements in your skin's appearance and your health.

Consistency is key; a regular bedtime routine will train your body to recognize when it's time to sleep, reducing the time it takes to fall asleep and minimizing disruptions during the night.

Different Eating Habits

What you eat can affect your skin's health. Nutrients from your diet help combat UV damage, improve skin elasticity, and reduce signs of aging.

Skin-Healthy Foods

- **Antioxidants**: Berries, nuts, and green leafy vegetables can help protect the skin from damage.
- **Healthy Fats**: Foods like avocados, salmon, and nuts provide essential fatty acids that keep your skin supple and moisturized.
- **Vitamins C and E**: Found in citrus fruits and seeds, these vitamins contribute to radiant skin and support the skin's natural repair system.

Adopting new eating habits can enhance skin health by nurturing the skin from the inside out. Nutritional changes can help manage inflammation, improve hydration, and boost your skin's natural glow.

Here are some dietary strategies that can impact skin health:

Intermittent Fasting

Intermittent fasting involves cycling between periods of eating and fasting. It can lead to improved metabolic health, reduction in oxidative stress, and better skin health. During fasting periods, the body initiates cellular repair processes, which can include autophagy, a process where cells clear out toxins and damaged components. For skin health, this may mean clearer and more youthful-looking skin due to reduced inflammation and enhanced ability to repair itself.

Reducing Carbohydrates

Lowering your intake of refined carbohydrates and sugars can decrease the production of insulin, which in turn reduces inflammation throughout the body. High levels of sugar in the diet can contribute to glycation, a process that can weaken the skin's collagen and elastin, leading to premature aging and loss of facial contour. By reducing these foods, you can enhance skin elasticity and reduce the formation of wrinkles.

Meal Prepping

Consistency is crucial for maintaining a healthy diet that supports skin health. Meal prepping involves planning and preparing meals in advance, ensuring that you have healthy options on hand throughout the week. This method helps maintain a balanced diet rich in fruits, vegetables, whole grains, and proteins—all vital for skin health. Eating a diet high in antioxidants, vitamins, and minerals supports collagen production, reduces inflammation, and shields the skin from damaging free radicals.

Implementing New Eating Habits

- **Plan Your Meals**: Start by planning a week's worth of meals that incorporate a variety of nutrients beneficial for skin health. Include plenty of antioxidants, healthy fats, and lean proteins (try meal delivery, too!).
- **Shop Smart**: Make a shopping list based on your meal plan that emphasizes fresh, unprocessed foods. Avoiding impulse buying of unhealthy foods begins with making informed choices at the grocery store.
- **Prepare in Batches**: Set aside time to cook meals in batches. This can save time during the week and make it easier to stick to your new eating habits without resorting to less healthy options.
- **Check Food Portion Sizes**: Be mindful of overeating. Proper portion control can help manage weight and reduce chronic inflammation, benefiting health and skin condition.

By adjusting what and how you eat, you can create a powerful impact on your skin's health and appearance. These changes enhance your wellness, providing a solid foundation for a healthy lifestyle.

Using Sunscreen

Protecting your skin from the sun is crucial at any age, but particularly after 50, as the skin becomes more susceptible to UV damage. Daily sunscreen use can prevent further age spots, wrinkles, and other skin damage.

- Apply a broad-spectrum sunscreen with at least SPF 30 daily, regardless of whether it's sunny or cloudy.
- Remember to apply every two hours if you are outdoors for extended periods.

Importance of Sunscreen

Regular use of sunscreen can reduce the accumulation of photodamage, maintaining the skin's integrity and youthful appearance. It is particularly vital as we age because mature skin becomes thinner and less resilient. Sunscreen acts as a shield, protecting vulnerable skin from further damage and reducing the risk of skin cancer.

Incorporating Sunscreen into the Morning Routine

Add sunscreen to your morning skincare routine. Apply it after moisturizer but before makeup. Allow the sunscreen to absorb and dry for a few minutes to form an effective barrier on the skin. For those who prefer a simpler routine, consider a moisturizer that already contains SPF. This combination product hydrates the skin while also providing UV protection, streamlining your skincare regimen.

Choosing the Right Sunscreen

When selecting a sunscreen, look for products offering broad-spectrum protection, which blocks both UVA and UVB rays. Use an SPF (sun protection factor) of at least 30 for daily use. Avoid sunscreens containing oxybenzone and octinoxate for their potential environmental risks, particularly to coral reefs, and may have hormonal effects in humans.

Organic vs. Chemical Sunscreens

Organic (or mineral) sunscreens contain active mineral ingredients, such as titanium dioxide or zinc oxide, which block UV radiation by sitting on top of the skin. These are often recommended for sensitive skin and are less likely to cause irritation. Chemical sunscreens, which absorb UV radiation through chemical reactions, can sometimes offer a lighter texture and less visible residue, making them preferable under makeup.

Benefits of Daily Sunscreen Use

- **Prevents Premature Aging**: Daily use helps maintain elasticity and reduce visible signs of aging caused by sun exposure.
- **Reduces Skin Cancer Risks**: Regular application lowers the risk of developing squamous cell carcinoma and melanoma.
- **Even Skin Tone**: Protects against discoloration and dark spots from sun damage.

Types of Sunscreen Available

- **Sunscreens Integrated in Moisturizers**: Ideal for daily use as they combine hydration with sun protection.
- **Mineral vs. Chemical Sunscreens**: Mineral sunscreens offer a physical barrier and are generally better for sensitive skin, while chemical sunscreens may be less noticeable once applied.
- **Tinted Sunscreens**: These provide light coverage for the skin while protecting it from the sun, serving as a dual-purpose product that can replace foundation.

By making sunscreen a non-negotiable part of your daily routine, you can enhance your skin's health and appearance, maintaining a youthful and vibrant look well into later years.

Drinking Water

Hydration is key to maintaining skin elasticity and moisture. Drinking adequate water throughout the day can help flush out toxins that may affect your skin's appearance.

By integrating these practices into your daily life, you can support your skin's health beyond your skincare products, contributing to a vibrant appearance. Staying hydrated is fundamental to maintaining healthy skin, particularly as we age. Water aids in maintaining skin elasticity and suppleness by replenishing skin tissues and increasing its moisture level. Understanding how much water to drink and how to incorporate it into your daily routine can enhance not your skin's appearance but your health.

Optimal Amount of Water

The amount of water an individual should drink can vary based on factors like age, weight, climate, and physical activity levels. Yet, a general rule of thumb is to aim for about 8-10 glasses (approximately 2 liters or half a gallon) of water per day. This guideline serves as a good baseline to ensure you're hydrated.

Incorporating More Water into Your Routine

- **Start Your Day with Water**: Drinking a glass of water first thing in the morning is a fantastic way to kickstart your hydration for the day. It helps to awaken your metabolism and hydrate your body after a night's sleep. Consuming water before any morning coffee or breakfast aids in maintaining optimal digestion and skin hydration.
- **Use a Measured Water Bottle**: Keeping a water bottle with measurements can help you track your intake throughout the day. Choose one that marks time intervals to keep your drinking on schedule.
- **Enhance Your Water**: Adding natural flavors such as slices of lemon, cucumber, or berries can make drinking water more enjoyable and refreshing. These additions not only improve taste but also contribute extra nutrients.
- **Drink Through a Straw**: Using a straw can often help you drink more water faster and more throughout the day. This is especially

useful if you are often busy and need to take quick sips.

Tips and Tricks to Increase Water Intake

- **Set Regular Reminders**: Use your phone or computer to set reminders to take a drink. Regular prompts can make a big difference in your daily water consumption.
- **Eat Water-Rich Foods**: Incorporate foods with high water content into your diet. Fruits like watermelon, strawberries, and cucumbers are tasty options that help increase your fluid intake.
- **Keep Water Accessible**: Always have a glass or bottle of water at your desk, in your car, or in your bag. Easy access to water increases the likelihood that you'll drink throughout the day.

Benefits of Drinking More Water

- **Enhanced Skin Health**: Adequate hydration helps to keep the skin moist and reduces the appearance of fine lines and wrinkles.
- **Improved Physical Performance**: Proper hydration contributes to optimal muscle function and energy levels.
- **Better Digestive Health**: Water is essential for good digestion and helps prevent constipation.
- **Detoxification**: Water helps to flush toxins from the body, supporting kidney function and promoting a healthy immune system.

Incorporating these practices into your daily routine can enhance your skin's health by ensuring that it is well-hydrated and functioning at its best. Remember, one key to beautiful skin could be as simple as drinking more water.

6

Conclusion

Remember, for women over 50, while these routines and tips are a great starting point, the unique needs of your skin may need personalized attention. Consulting with a dermatologist or esthetician can provide tailored advice, ongoing care, and insight into new products or treatments that might be beneficial for your skin type.

Each skin type presents its own challenges and benefits, but with the right care and advice, you can maintain a radiant and healthy complexion. Your renewed skincare is a journey, not a destination. It's about finding what works for you and adapting your routine as your skin's needs change over time.

This book aims to be a basic foundation providing knowledge and flexible approaches to help you look and feel your best. I hope you found the information helpful and it inspires you to embrace your skincare routine with confidence.

If you've enjoyed this book and found the tips beneficial, please consider leaving a positive review on Amazon. Your feedback supports my love for sharing practical information and helps others discover this book to enhance their skincare journey too!

Thank you for choosing my book, and here's to your continued skincare success!

♥

7

Resources

Cronkleton, E. (2020, May 12). *8 benefits of a facial massage*. Healthline. https://www.healthline.com/health/beauty-skin-care/facial-massage-benefits

Kadar, E. (2024, April 26). Best red light therapy devices for getting an at-home glow-up · AP Buyline Shopping. *AP Buyline Shopping*. https://apnews.com/buyline-shopping/article/best-red-light-therapy-devices

Keep your skin healthy. (2017, September 8). NIH News in Health. https://newsinhealth.nih.gov/2015/11/keep-your-skin-healthy

Millhone, C. (2023, October 30). *How to build a morning and evening skincare routine*. Health. https://www.health.com/skincare-routine-8364021

Msj, J. C. (2023, April 7). *The No BS guide to discovering your real skin type*. Healthline. https://www.healthline.com/health/beauty-skin-care/skin-type-test

Wang, S. (2024, May 5). Peptides vs. Retinoids Which is Best for Your Skin. *100% PURE*. https://www.100percentpure.com/blogs/feed/pepti des-vs-retinoids-which-is-best-for-your-skin

What to know about intermittent fasting for women after 50. (2021, September 27). WebMD. https://www.webmd.com/healthy-aging/ what-to-know-about-intermittent-fasting-for-women-after-50

OpenAI. (2023). ChatGPT. https://www.openai.com/chatgpt